Diagnosis and Treatment
of Sleep/Wake Disorders

D0109857

Every effort has been made in preparing this book to provide accurate and up-to-date information that is in accord with accepted standards and practice at the time of publication. Nevertheless, the author, editors, and publisher can make no warranties that the information contained herein is totally free from error, not least because clinical standards are constantly changing through research and regulation. The authors, editors, and publisher therefore disclaim all liability for direct or consequential damages resulting from the use of material contained in this book. Readers are strongly advised to pay careful attention to information provided by the manufacturer of any drugs or equipment that they plan to use.

PUBLISHED BY NEI PRESS, an imprint of NEUROSCIENCE EDUCATION INSTITUTE
Carlsbad, California, United States of America

NEUROSCIENCE EDUCATION INSTITUTE
1930 Palomar Point Way, Suite 101
Carlsbad, California 92008

http://www.neiglobal.com

Printed in the United States of America
First Edition, October 2007

Typeset in Futura

Library of Congress Cataloging-in-Publication Data
ISBN 1-4225-0017-9

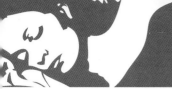

Table of Contents

CME Information

Overview
Sleep/wake disorders can cause significant impairment in social and work functioning due to their daytime effects on alertness, cognitive functioning, and mood. In this booklet we examine the underlying neurobiological causes of sleep/wake disorders as well as the current evidence and guidelines for diagnosis and treatment of patients presenting with these disorders.

Target Audience
This activity was designed for healthcare professionals, including psychiatrists, neurologists, primary care physicians, clinical psychologists, pharmacists, psychotherapists, nurses, nurse practitioners, addiction counselors, social workers and others, who treat patients with psychiatric conditions.

Statement of Need
The content of this educational activity was determined by rigorous assessment, including activity feedback, expert faculty assessment, and literature review, which revealed the following unmet needs:

- The neural circuitry implicated in the pathophysiology of sleep disorders is beginning to be understood
- Despite the well-established significant mental and physical health consequences of sleep disorders, they are under-recognized and under-treated
- Appropriate treatment options can differ depending on the cause of disordered sleep; in addition, for each sleep disorder there are multiple treatment options including pharmacological, behavioral, and others

Learning Objectives
Upon completion of this activity, you should be able to:

- Recognize underlying causes of sleep/wake disorders
- Identify patients for whom direct treatment of sleep/wake problems is necessary
- Effectively implement treatment plans for patients with sleep/wake disorders

Accreditation and Credit Designation Statements
The Neuroscience Education Institute is accredited by the Accreditation Council for Continuing Medical Education to provide continuing medical education for physicians.

The Neuroscience Education Institute designates this educational activity for a maximum of 2.5 *AMA PRA Category 1 Credits™*. Physicians should only claim credit commensurate with the extent of their participation in the activity.

Activity Instructions
This CME activity is in the form of a printed monograph and incorporates instructional design to enhance your retention of the information and pharmacological concepts that are being presented. You are advised to go through this activity from beginning to end and then complete the posttest and activity evaluation. The estimated time for completion of this activity is 2.5 hours.

Instructions for CME Credit
To receive your certificate of CME credit or participation, please complete the posttest (you must score at least 70% to receive credit) and activity evaluation found at the end of the monograph and mail or fax them to the address/number provided. Once received, your posttest will be graded and a certificate sent if a score of 70% or more was attained. Alternatively, you may complete the posttest and activity evaluation online and immediately print your certificate. There is no fee for this activity.

NEI Disclosure Policy
It is the policy of the Neuroscience Education Institute to ensure balance, independence,

objectivity, and scientific rigor in all its educational activities. The Neuroscience Education Institute takes responsibility for the content, quality, and scientific integrity of this CME activity.

All faculty participating in any NEI-sponsored educational activity and all individuals in a position to influence or control content development are required by NEI to disclose to the activity audience any financial relationships or apparent conflicts of interest that may have a direct bearing on the subject matter of the activity. Although potential conflicts of interest are identified and resolved prior to the activity, it remains for the audience to determine whether outside interests reflect a possible bias in either the exposition or the conclusions presented.

Individual Disclosure Statements

Authors/Developers
Meghan Grady
Director, Content Development
Neuroscience Education Institute, Carlsbad, CA
No other financial relationships to disclose.

Eleanor Roberts, MSc, PhD
Medical Writer
Neuroscience Education Institute, Carlsbad, CA
No other financial relationships to disclose.

Content Editor
Stephen M. Stahl, MD, PhD
Adjunct Professor, Department of Psychiatry
University of California, San Diego School of Medicine, San Diego, CA
Board Member: Cypress Bioscience; NeuroMolecular; Pierre Fabre; Tetragenix
Grant/Research: Alkermes; AstraZeneca; Bristol-Myers Squibb; Cephalon; Cyberonics; Eli Lilly; GlaxoSmithKline; Janssen; Jazz; Neurocrine Biosciences; Novartis; Organon; Pfizer; Sepracor; Shire; Somaxon; Takeda; Wyeth
Consultant/Advisor: Acadia; Amylin; AstraZeneca; Avera; Azur; Biovail; Boehringer Ingelheim; Bristol-Myers Squibb; Cephalon; CSC; Cyberonics; Cypress Bioscience; Eli Lilly; Epix; Forest; GlaxoSmithKline; Janssen; Jazz; Labopharm; Neurocrine Biosciences; NeuroMolecular; Neuronetics; Novartis; Organon; Pamlab; Pfizer; Pierre Fabre; sanofi-aventis; Schering-Plough; Sepracor; Shire; Solvay; Somaxon; Tethys; Tetragenix; Vanda; Wyeth
Speakers Bureau: AstraZeneca; Cephalon; CSC; Eli Lilly; Pfizer; Wyeth

Peer Reviewers
Meera Narasimhan, MD
Professor, Department of Psychiatry
Director of Biological Research, Office of Biological Research
Department of Neuropsychiatry and Behavioral Science
University of South Carolina School of Medicine, Columbia, SC
Grant/Research: AstraZeneca Pharmaceuticals LP; Bristol-Myers Squibb Company; Forest Laboratories, Inc.; Janssen Pharmaceutica Inc.
Consultant/Advisor: Bristol-Myers Squibb Company; Eli Lilly and Company
Speakers Bureau: AstraZeneca Pharmaceuticals LP; Bristol-Myers Squibb Company; Eli Lilly and Company; Janssen Pharmaceutica Inc.

Electa Stern, PharmD
Clinical Supervisor
Sharp Grossmont Hospital, La Mesa, CA
Attended Advisory Board: Aventis Pharmaceuticals Inc.; Johnson & Johnson; Novartis

Editorial & Design Staff
Rory Daley, MPH
Program Development Associate
Neuroscience Education Institute, Carlsbad, CA
No other financial relationships to disclose.

Stacey L. Hughes
Director, Program Development
Neuroscience Education Institute, Carlsbad, CA
No other financial relationships to disclose.

Nancy Muntner
Director, Medical Illustrations
Neuroscience Education Institute, Carlsbad, CA
No other financial relationships to disclose

Steve Smith
President and COO
Neuroscience Education Institute, Carlsbad, CA
No other financial relationships to disclose.

Jahon Jabali
Interactive Designer
Neuroscience Education Institute, Carlsbad, CA
No other financial relationships to disclose.

Disclosed financial relationships have been reviewed by the Neuroscience Education Institute CME Advisory Board to resolve any potential conflicts of interest. All faculty and planning committee members have attested that their financial relationships do not affect their ability to present well-balanced, evidence-based content for this activity.

Disclosure of Off-Label Use
This educational activity may include discussion of unlabeled and/or investigational uses of agents that are not approved by the FDA. Please consult the product prescribing information for full disclosure of labeled uses.

Disclaimer
Participants have an implied responsibility to use the newly acquired information from this activity to enhance patient outcomes and their own professional development. The information presented in this educational activity is not meant to serve as a guideline for patient management. Any procedures, medications, or other courses of diagnosis or treatment discussed or suggested in this educational activity should not be used by clinicians without evaluation of their patients' conditions and possible contraindications or dangers in use, review of any applicable manufacturer's product information, and comparison with recommendations of other authorities. Primary references and full prescribing information should be consulted.

Grantor Information
This activity is supported by an educational grant from Cephalon, Inc.

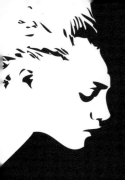

Neurobiology of Sleep/Wake

Chapter 1

Objectives

Apply an understanding of neurobiological and neurochemical mechanisms of arousal and sleep to the diagnosis of sleep/wake problems

Recognize that there is a spectrum of arousal, from hyperarousal to hypoarousal, which has been shown in a number of disorders but may stem from the same brain mechanisms

Recognize the role of the hypothalamic-pituitary-adrenal (HPA) axis in disorders of arousal and sleep

Identify the relationship between excessive sleepiness and problems such as vehicular accidents, medical errors, and work/school productivity

Excessive Sleepiness

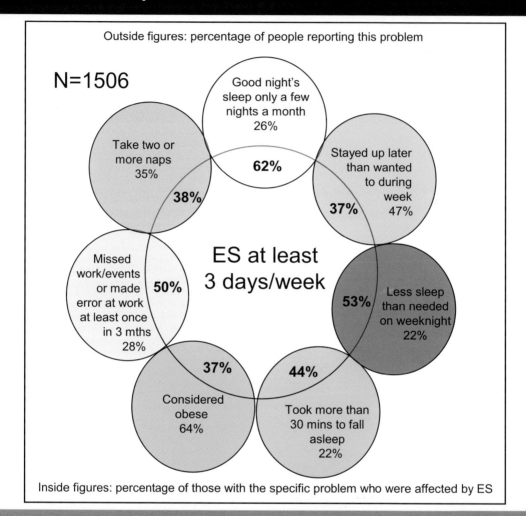

Outside figures: percentage of people reporting this problem

N=1506

Good night's sleep only a few nights a month 26%

62%

Take two or more naps 35%

38%

Stayed up later than wanted to during week 47%

37%

ES at least 3 days/week

Missed work/events or made error at work at least once in 3 mths 28%

50%

Less sleep than needed on weeknight 22%

53%

Considered obese 64%

37%

44%

Took more than 30 mins to fall asleep 22%

Inside figures: percentage of those with the specific problem who were affected by ES

Figure 1.1 In 2005, the National Sleep Foundation conducted a "Sleep in America Poll" that involved 1506 random telephone interviews with adults within the continental United States. Questions asked included the circumstances leading to excessive sleepiness (ES). These involved incidences of sleep disturbances such as getting less sleep than needed during the week, taking 30 minutes or more to fall asleep, and having to stay up later than wanted during the week. They found that one- to two-thirds of those who had these problems suffered from ES. For instance, of the 26% who said that they only got a good night's sleep a few nights a month, 62% also reported they had ES.

Problems with ES can affect a person's work and/or social life. Of the 28% who had missed work/events or made an error at work, half of them also suffered from ES. Of the physical factors examined, 62% considered themselves obese and of these over a third suffered from ES at least 3 days a week. A number of these factors will be considered in this booklet. [National Sleep Foundation, 2005]

Sleep and Arousal Pathways and Brain Regions

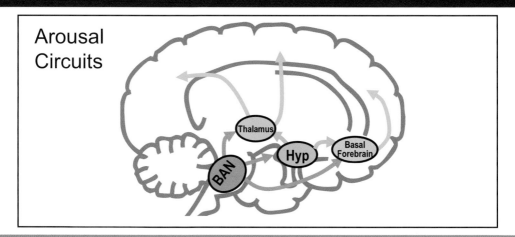

Figure 1.2 Most wake circuits originate in the brainstem arousal nuclei (BAN), which stimulate the thalamus, hypothalamus (Hyp) and basal forebrain. The hypothalamus itself stimulates the thalamus and basal forebrain, and these areas arouse the cortex. These projections also inhibit sleep centers such as those discussed below.

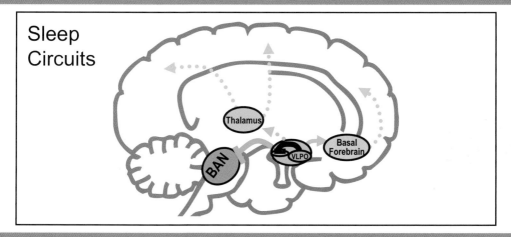

Figure 1.3 The ventrolateral preoptic nucleus (VLPO) in the hypothalamus inhibits the BAN and the parts of the hypothalamus involved in wakefulness. This leads to inhibition of other wake-centers including the thalamus, basal forebrain, and the cortex, and thus the initiation and maintenance of sleep. [Stenberg, 2007]

Hypothalamic Regulation of Sleep and Arousal

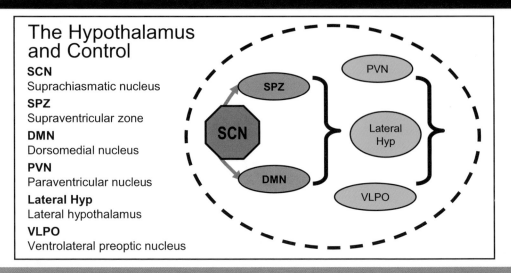

Figure 1.4 The sleep/wake cycle is controlled by distinct hypothalamic neurons. The SCN is the circadian "pacemaker" and is influenced by light, activity, and melatonin to promote either wake or sleep. Signals from the SCN are amplified by the SPZ and the DMN, which project to the VLPO (promotes sleep), the lateral hypothalamus (promotes wakefulness), and the PVN (controls pineal melatonin release).

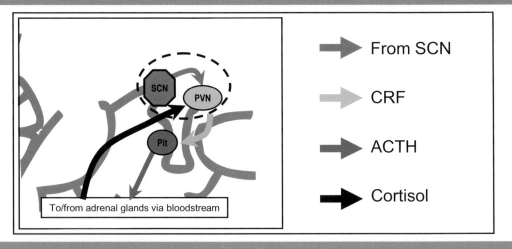

Figure 1.5 In the normal hypothalamic-pituitary-adrenal (HPA) axis, the PVN is stimulated by the SCN, in a circadian fashion, to produce corticotrophin-releasing factor (CRF). This acts on the pituitary gland (Pit), which in turn produces adrenocorticotrophic hormone (ACTH). ACTH is then released into the bloodstream where it initiates the release of cortisol from the adrenal glands. Cortisol is one of the factors involved in the sleep/wake cycle through a feedback system whereby it can then influence activity in the hypothalamus. Thus the HPA axis is important to regulation of sleep and arousal.

Circadian Rhythms and Wake Propensity

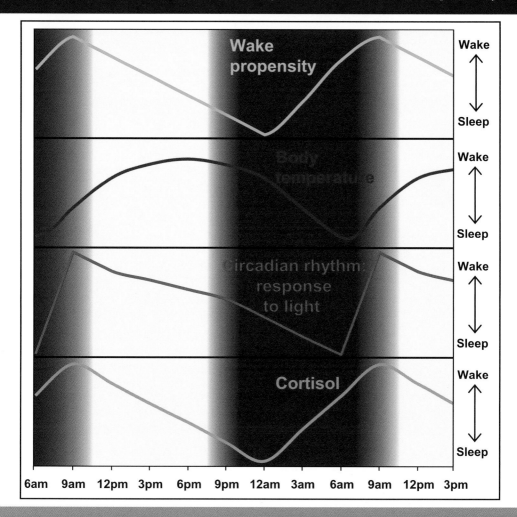

Figure 1.6 Several factors involved in the rhythmic control of sleep and wake are shown here. Circadian arousal is largely influenced by ocular exposure to light; thus it rises in the morning, declines with a gradual slope throughout the day, and then declines further beginning in the late evening. Body temperature is also at its lowest in the early morning, rising throughout the morning and then staying fairly steady until it begins to decline again in the late evening. Combined with this, a morning pulse of cortisol, which binds to circadian hypothalamic receptors, stimulates arousal from sleep with levels declining throughout the day. In addition, certain brain chemicals (e.g., adenosine, a byproduct of energy metabolism), accumulate during waking time and decline during sleep. The varying levels of these chemicals affect one's wake propensity, with wake propensity declining as they accumulate and then increasing as the sleep debt is paid. [Saper et al., 2005; Dijk and Lockley, 2002]

The Arousal Spectrum

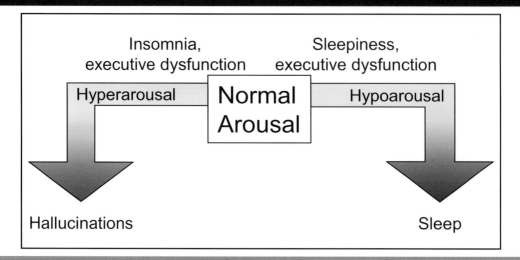

Figure 1.7 Whether we are asleep or awake depends on the interaction between many key players: circadian rhythms, ultradian cycles, and homeostatic drive. However, "awake" and "asleep" are not the only states of arousal; rather, arousal is akin to a dimmer switch that affects a person's behavior depending on how high or low the switch is turned.

Hyperarousal is considered an underlying cause of insomnia and may be related to dysfunction of the HPA axis. Specifically, HPA dysfunction can lead to increases in CRF and cortisol release. These factors feed back to cause additional activation of both the HPA axis and arousal systems, such as the locus coeruleus, during the night. Thus, during hyperarousal arousal circuits fail to turn off, and whole-brain metabolism remains more akin to the waking than the sleeping state. Problems arising from this hyperarousal include sleep fragmentation and a decrease of the more "refreshing" slow-wave sleep. In extreme cases of hyperarousal, individuals may even experience hallucinations.

With hypoarousal, there is thought to be reduced basal ACTH secretion and a reduction of central CRF. Extreme hypoarousal underlies excessive sleepiness present in numerous sleep/wake disorders, which is the focus of this booklet and is discussed in more detail later.

Ailments along the trajectory connecting both extremes are more intriguing and their treatment can be controversial. Mild sleepiness, regardless of cause, may lead to executive dysfunction. Similarly, being in a state of hyperarousal, even mild hyperarousal, can impair cognitive functioning. Thus the question remains, is there a relationship between sleep/wake disorders and cognitive disorders? Sleep circuits overlap with many neurobiological circuits underlying cognitive functioning, as discussed in more detail on the following page. [Buckley and Schatzberg, 2005]

Disordered Sleep Affects Executive Function

Circuit	Function	Lesion
DLPFC	Problem Solving Cognitive Flexibility Self Monitoring Planning	↓ Working Memory ↓ Attention ↓ Organizational Skills
OFC	Sensory Integration Response Inhibition Emotional Regulation	↑ Impulsivity ↑ Distractibility ↑ Disordered Behavior
ACC	Goal-Directed Behavior Error Processing Emotional Output Attention	↓ Error Monitoring ↓ Stroop Performance

Figure 1.8 Symptoms of sleepiness can affect daily life, including our higher executive functions. This is because circuits involving sleep centers can overlap with those controlling attentional processes. The main pathways involved in attention are the ascending projections from catecholaminergic nuclei in the brainstem, and from cholinergic cells of the basal forebrain to the prefrontal cortex. These are the same nuclei that are important in maintaining cortical arousal.

In general, the dorsolateral prefrontal cortex (DLPFC) is involved in problem solving, cognitive flexibility, self monitoring and planning. Lesions here can lead to problems with working memory, attention, and organization skills.

The orbitofrontal cortex (OFC) is involved in the mediation of information about the internal environment, including sensory signals, as well as inhibiting inappropriate responses and regulating emotional behavior. Lesions here can lead to impulsivity, distractibility, disordered behavior, and difficulties in responding appropriately to social cues.

The anterior cingulate cortex (ACC) mediates goal-directed behavior, partly by aiding the selection of internally relevant cues to environmental situations; monitors conflict situations; helps control emotional output; and is involved in the voluntary allocation of attention. Studies of lesion here show sufferers responding less to errors and performance deficits on cognitive tests. [Arnsten, 2005; Heyder, 2004; Shipp, 2004]

Consequences of Sleep Deprivation

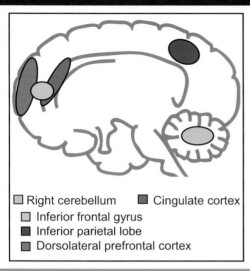

□ Right cerebellum   ■ Cingulate cortex
□ Inferior frontal gyrus
■ Inferior parietal lobe
■ Dorsolateral prefrontal cortex

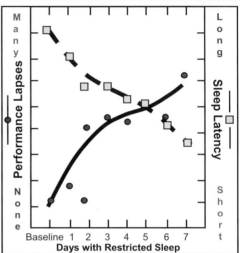

Figure 1.9 In the short-term, sleep deprivation can be compensated for and people who have had little to no sleep can function somewhat normally in everyday tasks.

As an example, Drummond et al. (2005) used a word memorizing task and showed that when recalling easy to learn words, sleep deprived subjects reported finding the task slightly more difficult but showed no difference in brain activation compared to after a normal night's sleep. However, when asked to memorize and recall hard to learn words there were significant increases in brain activation in the regions shown in color above.

As performance levels did not change it was thus shown that to be able to complete a task at the same level as normal the sleep deprived brain has to both increase activation in the regions usually utilized in this task and recruit additional brain regions. It is of note that activation and recruitment during the harder task was found in many of the brain regions previously discussed as being involved in executive functioning. [Drummond et al., 2005]

Figure 1.10 In the "real world" it is more often the case that sleep is below average (not totally deprived) over an extended period of time. Dinges et al. (1997) restricted sleep to an average 4.98 hours per night over 7 days. The results were that cumulative sleep debt produced significant problems with fatigue, confusion, tension, and total mood disturbance; in addition, psychomotor vigilance generally decreased day by day. Interestingly, overall changes in these measures were great during the first 2 days, recovered slightly during the next 3 days, and then fell again during the last 2 days.

This shows that it is possible for the body and brain to compensate for sleep deprivation in the short-term, but that if this continues it can "run out" of resources. In addition, sleepiness and performance problems continued for around 2 days after the end of the study, despite participants having a normal sleep time. The graph above combines the results of this study showing performance deficits with the effect of sleep deprivation on sleep latency during the day. [Dinges et al., 1997]

Consequences of Untreated Symptoms: Vehicular Accidents

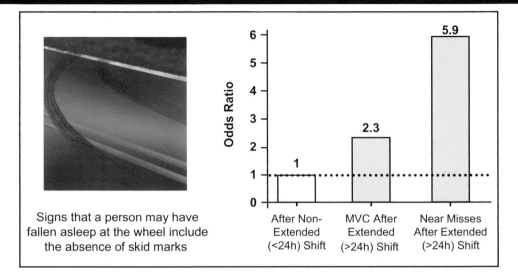

Signs that a person may have fallen asleep at the wheel include the absence of skid marks

Figure 1.11 In the 2005 Sleep in America Poll, 37% of the respondents who "drive or have a license" said that they have, at some point in their lives, nodded off or fallen asleep while driving. 5% said that this occurs at least once a month and 4% said they have had an accident or near accident in the past year because of dozing or being too tired while driving.

During accident investigations a key sign that someone has drifted off behind the wheel is the absence of tire skid marks or signs of hard braking such as could be shown on a truck driver's tachograph. Many drivers who have had a sleep-related vehicle accident (SRVA) cannot recollect falling asleep, and, indeed, it has been found in sleep studies that people who fall asleep for less than two minutes generally do not recall it.

The peak time of SRVAs is 02:00–06:00 and 14:00–16:00, coinciding with the circadian lows. The biggest sector of people who have SRVAs are those who drive company cars and trucks, especially at night; drivers who are on call for extended periods; people who have long work hours; and those driving home from a night shift.

A study of medical interns showed that the odds ratio of having a "near miss" during the commute home from work was 5.9 times higher following a shift lasting more than 24 hours, and having an actual motor vehicle crash (MVC) was 2.3 times higher. It was also found that for every extra extended shift per month the risk of a crash on the commute from work increased by 16.2%. Additionally, the odds ratios for falling asleep behind the wheel significantly increased with the number of extended shifts worked per month. [Horne and Reyner, 1999; Barger, 2005]

Consequences of Untreated Symptoms: Medical Errors and School Achievement

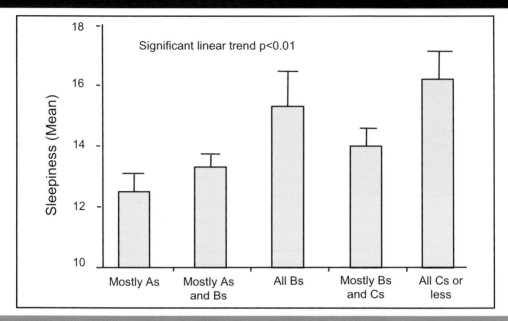

Figure 1.12 Excessive sleepiness can significantly impair performance and increase the risk of errors. When a child or adolescent's grades start slipping, parents and teachers often overlook sleep problems as a causative factor. Drake et al. (2003) looked at 442 students (aged 11 to 15 years) and found a significant linear relationship between ES and total sleep time as well as between Pediatric Daytime Sleepiness Scale (PDSS) scores and school achievement, anger towards self and others, and more frequent illness.

Adolescents' circadian rhythms can be shifted such that they cannot get to sleep until late, and want to wake up later as well. This study also showed that over two-thirds of eighth graders, compared to just over one-third of sixth graders, reported bedtimes of 11:00pm or later, and that over double the percentage of eighth graders (40%) reported getting less than 7 hours sleep on school nights. Accordingly, PDSS score increased with grade level. This circadian shift and an adolescent's need for more than 8 hours sleep a night is now being recognized by some schools who are experimenting with later school start times.

Increased work errors as a result of excessive sleepiness can be a safety concern. Suzuki (2005) surveyed hospital nurses about occupational accidents due to excessive sleepiness (ES). Over a quarter of nurses answered "yes" to the question, "Do you feel excessively sleepy during the daytime?" and nearly half said that their sleep sufficiency was "very insufficient" or "insufficient."

For those who had an error when administering a drug, the incident was associated with ES, sleep medication use, age, and night or irregular shift work, the last being significantly correlated. Incorrect operation of medical equipment also showed significant associations with ES and age (those over 50). This study suggests that there is a correlation between medical errors and ES, especially for nurses working irregular shifts and/or night shifts. [Drake et al. 2003; Suzuki, 2005]

Summary

People can suffer from excessive sleepiness for a number of reasons.

During the day arousal circuits normally inhibit sleep circuits, with a role reversal during the night.

Many sleep-related problems involve and affect the same neurobiological systems even if they do not stem from the same neurobiological systems.

There is a "spectrum of arousal" from hyperarousal to sleep which can all be associated with sleep-related problems.

The HPA axis is intimately involved in arousal and sleep and disruptions can lead to either hyperarousal or hypoarousal.

Problems with hyper- and hypoarousal can affect executive functions and, therefore, performance.

While short-term sleep deprivation may be compensated for, long-term sleep restriction can affect psychomotor and cognitive performance.

Consequences of untreated excessive sleepiness can include vehicular accidents, medical errors, decreased work productivity/school achievement, and/or increased psychiatric symptoms.

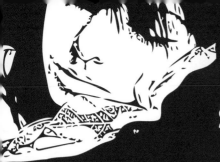

Diagnosing
Sleep/Wake Disorders

Chapter 2

Objectives

Gain knowledge of the tests for investigation of sleep/wake problems to help in diagnosis

Understand the underlying biological factors involved in narcolepsy, obstructive sleep apnea, shift-work sleep disorder, restless legs syndrome, and periodic limb movements of sleep

Diagnose and distinguish sleep/wake disorders in order to provide effective treatment and improve patient outcomes

Polysomnography (PSG)

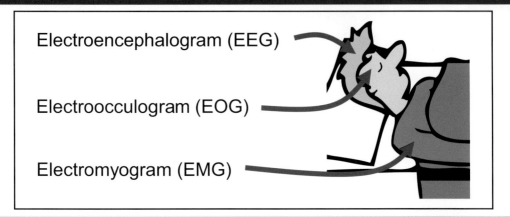

Figure 2.1 PSG may be used when certain sleep/wake disorders are suspected, such as periodic limb movement disorder (PLMD), narcolepsy, or obstructive sleep apnea (OSA). During PSG, an EEG is used to determine which sleep stage a person is in, an EOG measures eye movement to identify rapid eye movement sleep, and an EMG measures muscle movement via electrodes on the chin, jaw bone, and calf muscles.

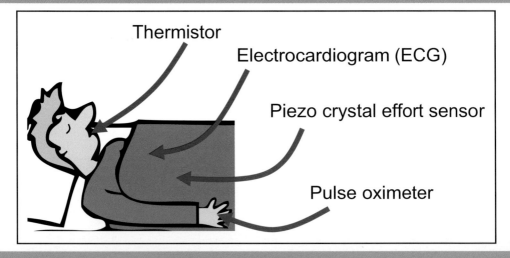

Figure 2.2 In addition, an electrocardiogram (ECG) is used to measure heart rate and rhythm, and breathing is measured with a piezo crystal effort sensor, which utilizes two Velcro bands around the chest and abdomen to measure movements and effort. Airflow is measured with a "thermistor" secured under the nose and oxygen saturation can be measured by a "pulse oximeter" on the finger or ear lobe. Finally the patient may also be videotaped. [Meir et al., 2005]

Tests of Wakefulness and Sleepiness

Maintenance of Wakefulness Test (MWT)

- Quiet, secure, comfortable temperature, low light that allows patient to focus on objects in the room, but not too bright
- Patient in a comfortable sitting position, with a back support
- Patient in daytime clothing
- Instructed to
  - "Sit and remain still, try and stay awake for as long as you can without extreme measures"
- Four attempted naps at 2-hour intervals beginning around 10:00am
- Sleep latency measured as time from beginning of trial to the first epoch at any sleep stage
- Nap is terminated as soon as sleep onset is recognized

Multiple Sleep Latency Test (MSLT)

- Dark, comfortable room at an ambient temperature
- Smoking, stimulants and vigorous physical activity avoided during the day, only light breakfast and lunch given
- Instructions are to
  - "Lie quietly in comfy position, keep eyes closed, try to fall asleep"
- Five nap opportunities at 2 hour intervals—initial nap opportunity 1.5–3 hours after termination of usual sleep
- Between naps patient out of bed and awake
- Sleep onset determined by time from "lights out" to first epoch of any sleep stage
- To assess occurrence of REM sleep the test continues for 15 minutes from first sleep epoch
- Session terminated if sleep does not occur after 20 minutes

Figures 2.3 and 2.4 The Maintenance of Wakefulness Test and the Multiple Sleep Latency Test are carried out in sleep laboratories, often after a night of PSG and a week filling in a sleep diary. As there are different mechanisms for arousal maintenance and sleep induction, these tests can measure different aspects of excessive sleepiness. Association between scores on these two measures is not uniform across disorders, and thus sleep studies should involve both measures. [Sangal et al., 1992]

Epworth Sleepiness Scale

Likelihood of falling asleep or dozing off when:	Chance of Dozing			
Sitting and reading	0	1	2	3
Watching television	0	1	2	3
Sitting inactive in a public place—theatre, meeting	0	1	2	3
As a car passenger for an hour without a break	0	1	2	3
Lying down to rest in the afternoon	0	1	2	3
Sitting and talking to someone	0	1	2	3
Sitting quietly after lunch without alcohol	0	1	2	3
Stopped for a few minutes while driving a car	0	1	2	3
Total Score				

Likelihood scale—rate each from 0–3 and total score

0—Would never doze
1—Slight chance of dozing
2—Moderate chance of dozing
3—High chance of dozing

Score over 11 indicates abnormal sleepiness

Figure 2.5 The Epworth Sleepiness Scale (ESS) is a self-rating tool to enable patients and physicians to easily investigate problems with excessive sleepiness. For the most part it can be used both for looking at a day as a whole or for various times throughout a person's wake time to chart their circadian changes. As a self-rating tool, it is of course subjective, and may not correlate well with objective test measures.

For the general population, the average score on the ESS may be approximately 5.9; scores over 11 indicate excessive sleepiness. Interestingly, those with insomnia may have scores lower than the general population, lending further weight to the theory that insomnia is a disorder of the arousal mechanisms that, as well as keeping someone awake at night, can leave someone in a state of hyperarousal during the day. [Stahl, in press]

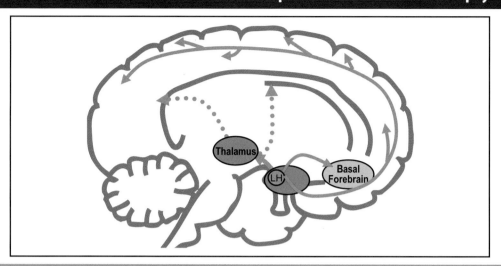

Figure 2.6 Orexin/hypocretin (Orx) is released predominantly while awake and is important in general arousal. Orexin is thought to suppress REM sleep and increase the excitatory tone of arousal circuits. Although orexin neurons are only found in a small population of cells in the lateral hypothalamus (LH), they have wide ranging projections.

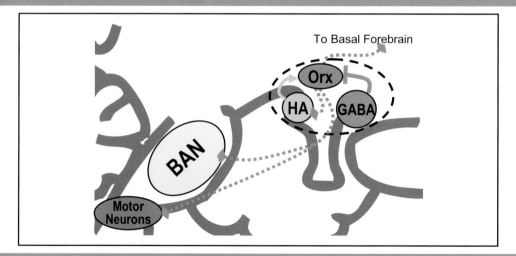

Figure 2.7 Orexin neurons have reciprocal projections to hypothalamic histamine (HA) neurons, as well as to the brainstem arousal neurons (BAN), motor neurons, and the basal forebrain. In narcolepsy there is a deficiency in orexin leading to rapid destabilization of the arousal circuits and thus extreme and sudden sleepiness. In addition, there may be a lack of stimulation to motor neurons, which can cause cataplexy, or loss of muscle tone. [Scammell, 2003]

Diagnosis of Narcolepsy

International Classification of Sleep Disorders
Diagnostic Criteria of Narcolepsy

- Patient complains of excessive sleepiness or sudden muscle weakness
- Recurrent daytime naps or lapses into sleep almost daily for at least 3 months
- Possible sleep-onset REM periods, hypnagogic hallucinations, and sleep paralysis
- With cataplexy
  - Sudden bilateral loss of postural muscle tone in association with intense emotion
- Hypersomnia not better explained by another disorder
- Should be confirmed by PSG followed by MSLT which should show a mean sleep latency of <8 minutes and two or more sleep-onset REM periods (SOREMPs) following normal sleep
- May be confirmed by orexin levels in the cerebrospinal fluid <110 pg/ml or <1/3 of mean normal control levels

Figure 2.8 Narcolepsy is estimated to occur in 0.03–0.16% of the general population, with its development mostly beginning in the teens. Narcoleptic sleep attacks usually occur for 10–20 minutes and, on awakening, the patient can be refreshed for 2–3 hours before feeling the need to sleep again. Although sleep attacks occur most often in monotonous situations, they can also occur when a person is actively conversing or eating. Symptoms of narcolepsy may include frightening hypnagogic hallucinations and sleep paralysis, which are usually coincident with SOREMPs. Not everyone with narcolepsy will have cataplexy but it is a unique feature of this disorder. An attack normally lasts a few seconds to minutes, during which the person is conscious. Some people have only minimal muscle involvement, while others can have "full-body" attacks; however, the respiratory and ocular muscles are never involved. Excessive sleepiness is the main symptom to continue with age, and it may worsen alongside the development of periodic limb movements and obstructive sleep apnea. In addition, sleep may be disrupted and include frequent awakenings. [ICSD rev, 2001]

Diagnosis of Obstructive Sleep Apnea

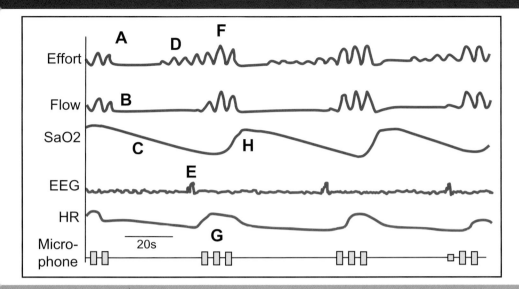

Figure 2.9 Obstructive sleep apnea (OSA) is most common in middle-aged people with a high BMI, a large neck circumference, and/or an underlying upper airway obstruction. It has an estimated prevalence of 4% for men and 2% for women. The diagnostic criteria for OSA include complaints of excessive sleepiness and/or difficulty sleeping as well as frequent episodes of obstructed breathing during sleep that may lead to awakening with breath holding, gasping or choking. Associated features include snoring, morning headache, and dry mouth on wakening.

Diagnosis of OSA should be carried out in a sleep laboratory using PSG. Detailed above is a number of readings that would be expected to be seen. A) The pharyngeal muscles collapse at the beginning of an apneic event (effort), leading to B) zero airflow (flow) and C) a drop in oxygen saturation (SaO2) (which can be to below 50%). This is followed by D), an increase in respiratory effort, E) an arousal reaction, as shown on the EEG, and F) an increase in pharyngeal muscle tone, leading to the upper airways opening again, hyperventilation, accompanied by G) snoring (microphone), and tachycardia. These events lead to a recovery period as can be seen with H) a return to normal oxygen saturation. Apneic episodes normally last for 20–40 seconds, most often during REM sleep and sleep stages 1 and 2. They can be followed by loud snores and vocalizations, as well as whole-body movements and microarousals.

Upon awakening patients can feel unrefreshed, disoriented, groggy, and uncoordinated. These problems can be accompanied by a severe dry mouth and a dull, generalized headache. The presenting complaint of those found to have OSA is predominantly excessive sleepiness, although unexplained depression, anxiety, and irritability often accompany OSA. Mild hypotension with an elevated diastolic pressure is also commonly associated with OSA and bradytachycardia can accompany an apneic event and can increase the risk of sudden death. [ICSD rev, 2001; Gilmartin et al., 2005]

Consequences of Obstructive Sleep Apnea

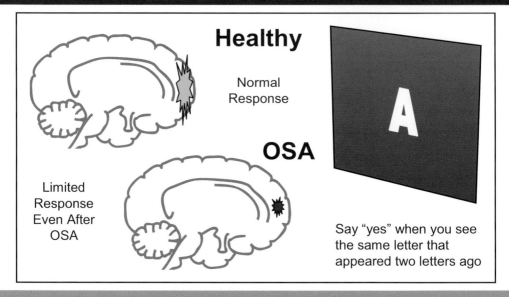

Figure 2.10 Occurrence of OSA can interfere with prefrontal cortical executive functions including attention, concentration, alertness, and memory, as well as physical measures such as reaction time. These may be due not only to the consequences of sleep fragmentation from an apneic episode, but also to the intermittent hypoxemia and hypercarbia that the apnea can cause. Other problems that may stem from these factors include poor motivation and increased chances of developing an affective disorder.

Thomas et al. (2005) used the 'n-back' test where subjects are shown a series of items/numbers/letters and are told to respond whenever an item matches another item shown 'n' (in this case 2) items ago. This task was used to investigate working memory, specifically through activation of the DLPFC, in patients with OSA compared to a group of control subjects.

The study showed that while in the control group there was activation of the DLPFC during the n-back test, there was almost an absence of activation in this area in the patients with OSA. This was regardless of whether the OSA patients suffered from nocturnal hypoxia, and despite the fact that the percentage of correct responses was high. Although, clinically, patients recovered following the use of continuous positive airway pressure (CPAP) therapy (which will be discussed later), the decrease in DLPFC activation remained. [Thomas et al., 2005]

Factors Underlying Shift-Work Sleep Disorder

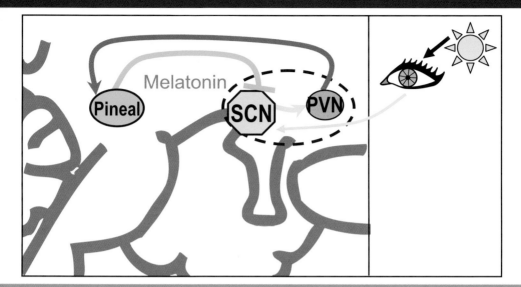

Figure 2.11 The main factors controlling the circadian rhythm of arousal are light, melatonin, and activity. Retinal receptors project to the SCN, which also receives information from the pineal gland, mostly via melatonin. This release of melatonin is indirectly controlled by the SCN through the PVN and via the brainstem.

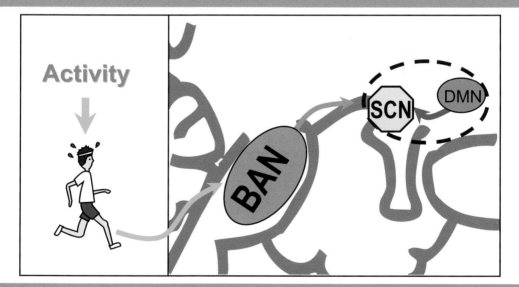

Figure 2.12 Information about the body's activity state is conveyed to the SCN through indirect projections from the brainstem arousal nuclei (BAN). There is also local feedback inhibition from other hypothalamic areas, such as the dorsomedial nucleus (DMN). [Saper et al., 2005; Mistlberger, 2005]

Shift-Work Sleep Disorder

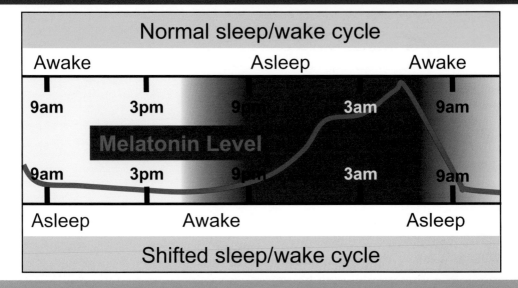

Figure 2.13 Up to 5% of adults are thought to suffer from shift-work sleep disorder and this can lead not only to reduced work productivity, errors, and vehicular accidents, but also to mood problems such as irritability, malaise, hostility, and depression.

While some people find that their circadian rhythm shifts to match their daily/nightly activity, those who suffer from shift-work sleep disorder are not able to adjust to the mismatch between their normal circadian sleep-wake pattern and the pattern required by that person's environment. This can lead to daytime insomnia, due to the arousal centers being normally activated by light, and nighttime excessive sleepiness.

The diagnosis of shift-work sleep disorder generally begins with a detailed patient history including questions such as:

Do you . . .

    Feel irritable or sleepy during your shift?
    Fall asleep sometimes while driving?
    Have difficulty paying attention, concentrating, and/or working to your full potential?
    Get told by others that you look tired?
    Have emotional outbursts?
    Feel like taking a nap while working?
    Require caffeinated beverages throughout the night to keep yourself going?

This should be followed by a 7-day sleep diary and may include the wearing of a sleep actigraph, a watch-like device that records gross activity. [Schwartz, 2006]

**Restless Legs Syndrome (RLS) and
Periodic Limb Movements (PLMs)**

Cardinal Diagnostic Features of RLS

1) Urge to move limbs usually associated with paresthesias or dysesthesias
2) Symptoms start or become worse with rest
3) At least partial relief with physical activity
4) Worsening of symptoms in the evening or at night

Figure 2.14 Patients with RLS experience an urge to move their legs to rid themselves of unpleasant sensations (prickling, tingling, burning, or tickling; numbness; "pins and needles"; or cramp-like sensations). This movement typically relieves the sensations, which can occur at any time but are most disruptive when one is trying to fall asleep.

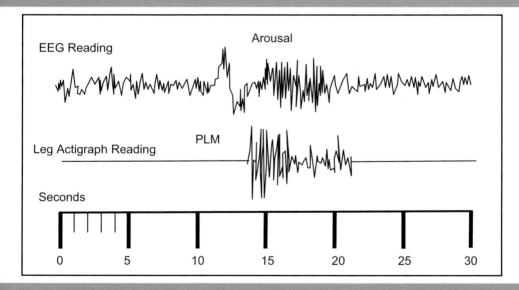

Figure 2.15 PLMs are involuntary movements that can occur during sleep or when awake. Muscle activation usually occurs in a sequence of 0.5–15 second contractions at intervals of 5–90 seconds and may arouse a person from sleep. Up to 87% with RLS will have PLMs but not everyone with PLMs has RLS. Diagnosis must involve an overnight electromyogram to distinguish PLM from other involuntary sleep movements [ICSD rev, 2001; Gilmartin et al., 2005]

Neurobiology of RLS and PLMs

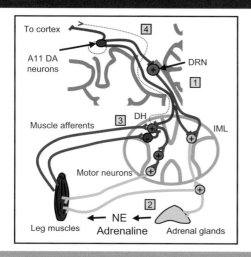

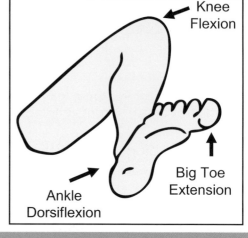

Figure 2.16 The prevalence of RLS ranges from 3–15% and increases with age. It is two times greater in women and is also familial.

The proposed cause is shown above: 1) inhibitory actions of A11 dopamine (DA) neurons are compromised, allowing the excitatory serotonergic dorsal raphe nucleus (DRN) projections to dominate in the spinal cord. 2) An increase in sympathetic drive can result in increased norepinephrine (NE) and adrenal gland released adrenaline, which leads to aberrant activation of high-threshold muscle afferents. 3) Loss of DA inhibitory controls in the region relaying high-threshold deep afferent input to the brain also leads to enhanced and aberrant signaling of ascending transmission of HTMAs. 4) The resulting focal akathisia may be exacerbated by a compromised A11 modulatory control of higher order sensory processing.

It is thought that the proximity of A11 cells to the hypothalamus explains the circadian nature of RLS and that, as dopamine production requires ferritin, inadequate iron stores/abnormal metabolism may decrease brain dopamine production and contribute to RLS. [Meir et al., 2005]

Figure 2.17 Although around 80% of people with RLS also have PLMs, it is thought to arise from a separate mechanism and can be experienced with or without RLS.

The action of PLMs consists of extension of the big toes, ankle dorsiflexion and, occasionally, flexion of the knee and hip, occurring every 20–40 seconds. It predominantly occurs at the beginning of the sleep cycle, where general periodic arousals are most common, and mostly disappears during deep sleep and REM sleep. PLMs are associated with tachycardia, tachypnoea, and increases in systemic blood pressure, all of which can lead to arousal from sleep and thus disruptions in daytime functioning.

Although it is unclear whether PLMs start in the limbs or are generated within spinal cord neurons, it is known that the timing of PLMs is modulated by descending influences and the current view is that the brainstem is the common trigger. [Vetrugno et al., 2007]

Summary

There are a number of measures designed to identify sleep/wake problems which may involve a simple rating scale or a visit to a sleep clinic.

Narcolepsy is a disorder involving lack of hypothalamic orexin, which affects motor and brainstem neurons.

Narcolepsy diagnosis, which does not necessarily include cataplexy, should involve assessment at a sleep clinic.

OSA follows a characteristic series of events that can lead to multiple awakenings; consequences of OSA include excessive sleepiness, depression, irritability, and cognitive dysfunction.

Our circadian rhythm is most influenced by daylight, which can be counteractive in those with SWSD.

Diagnosis of SWSD is generally through a detailed patient history and a sleep diary.

RLS and PLMs both have unelucidated etiologies.

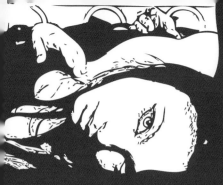

Treatment of Sleep/Wake Disorders

Chapter 3

Objectives

Advise patients on appropriate sleep hygiene practices in order to alleviate symptoms associated with sleep deprivation

Differentiate mechanisms of action for medications used in the treatment of sleep/wake disorders

Implement appropriate management strategies for patients with sleep/wake disorders in order to improve patient outcomes

Sleep/Wake Hygiene

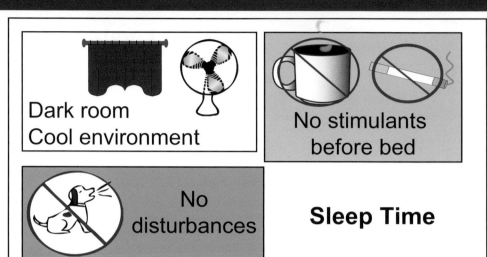

Figure 3.1 Difficulty falling or staying asleep can often be caused or exacerbated by poor sleep hygiene. Using caffeine, exercising, working, or doing stimulating things late in the evening; having a room that is too hot/cold or too light; having outside disturbances (e.g., noisy neighbors, disruptive pets); or keeping an inconsistent sleep/wake schedule should always be examined first.

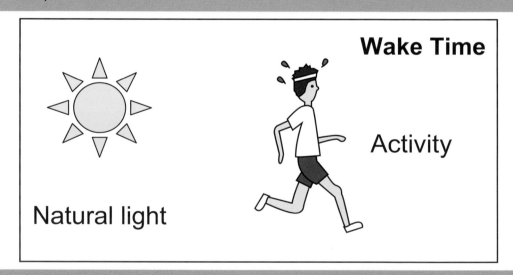

Figure 3.2 During a person's wake time excessive sleepiness can be exacerbated by being inside, without natural light, and being sedentary. Therefore both sunlight and activity can help relieve or prevent excessive sleepiness.

Treatment Guidelines

	Modafinil	Methylphenidate (d,l)	Methylphenidate (d)	Amphetamines	Caffeine	Sodium oxybate	Melatonin	Sleep aids	Ropinirole	Pramipexole	Antidepressants
Narcolepsy: sleepiness	X	X	X	X	X	X					
Narcolepsy: cataplexy						X					X
OSA: sleepiness	X	X	X	X	X						
Shift-work sleep disorder	X	X	X	X	X		X	X			
RLS/PLM	X	X	X	X				X	X	X	
Idiopathic hypersomnia	X	X	X	X	X						

Figure 3.3 For the most part, the same pharmacologic options can be used to treat ES regardless of a patient's diagnosis, as shown in the chart above (green denotes FDA approval for the specified indication). Thus, methylphenidate, amphetamines, or modafinil can be used to treat ES in narcolepsy, OSA, circadian rhythm disorders, restless legs syndrome, periodic limb movement disorder, or idiopathic hypersomnia, as well as to treat ES associated with medical or psychiatric conditions. Sodium oxybate, though it is efficacious for ES, has a difficult dosing schedule and would likely not be a preferred choice for patients who do not also have cataplexy. Each of these medications is examined in turn on the following pages, focusing on mechanism of action, dosing, and side effects.

Beyond ES, treatment for sleep/wake disorders will likely vary based on the underlying neurobiological basis for the symptoms, as indicated in the chart above. More specific treatment recommendations for the sleep/wake disorders shown here are covered later in this chapter. [Erman, 2006]

Treating Excessive Sleepiness: Methylphenidate

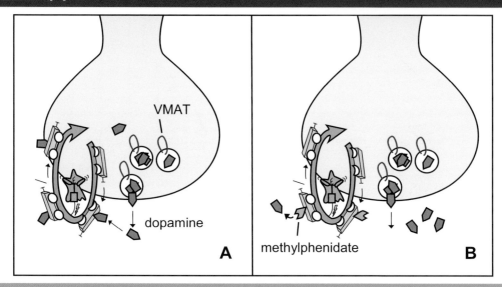

Figure 3.4 Psychostimulant-induced arousal is dependent on the actions of dopamine, along with norepinephrine, within both the prefrontal cortex, the limbic areas, and a network of subcortical regions. Following dopamine release, this neurotransmitter is taken back into the neuron by the dopamine transporter (DAT) and once inside the cell can be stored again in synaptic vesicles via the actions of the vesicular transporter (VMAT) (A). Methylphenidate prevents dopamine reuptake by binding to the DAT (B).

Functional imaging studies have shown that methylphenidate can increase frontal activation in people with intact functioning. Activation induced by methylphenidate here, as well as in the cerebellum and frontal temporal cortex, is significantly correlated with dopamine D2 receptor availability, thus responses to psychostimulants are determined in part by the working of the dopamine system.

Methylphenidate is available in a racemic form (d,l), of which there are many formulations which vary in terms of release (immediate release Ritalin, Methylin, generic; sustained release Ritalin SR, Methylin SR, Metadate ER, generic; time release beads Metadate CD; SODAS microbeads Ritalin LA; OROS Concerta). Methylphenidate is also available as the d-enantiomer (immediate and extended release Focalin). Immediate release formulations are recommended for excessive sleepiness, dosed 2–3 times per day for a total daily dose of 20–60 mg (racemic) or 5–20 mg (d-enantiomer). Notable side effects include insomnia, headache, nervousness, irritability, overstimulation, tremor, and dizziness. Methylphenidate has high abuse potential and is Schedule II, with greater risk for immediate release formulations, although methylphenidate may be less reinforcing than amphetamines. [Stahl, in press; Stahl, 2005]

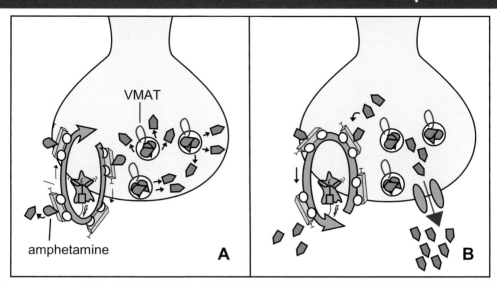

Figure 3.5 Amphetamine, like methylphenidate, binds to the DAT and prevents it from taking up dopamine. However, it is also itself taken up into the neuron where it binds the vesicular transporter (VMAT) (A). Competitive inhibition of amphetamine with dopamine at the VMAT leads to transport of amphetamine into the synaptic vesicles, which in turn causes displacement of dopamine from synaptic vesicles, intracellular dopamine accumulation, channel opening, and dopamine release into the synapse. It also causes a reversal of DAT function, so that dopamine is pumped out of the neuron instead of into it (B).

Amphetamines are available as the d-enantiomer (immediate and sustained release Dexedrine) and as the racemic (immediate and extended release Adderall). Like methylphenidate, dosing of amphetamines for excessive sleepiness is recommended at 20–60 mg/day divided into 2–3 doses. The side effects are also similar and include insomnia, headache, nervousness, irritability, overstimulation, tremor, and dizziness. Like methylphenidate, amphetamines are Schedule II drugs. There is a subtly greater dopamine release by amphetamines than methylphenidate in the prefrontal cortex, which is thought to account for the subtle differences in effects of these drugs on behavioral tolerance. [Stahl, in press; Stahl, 2005]

Treating Excessive Sleepiness: Modafinil

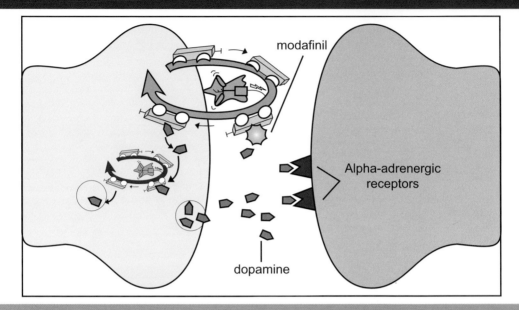

Figure 3.6 The precise mechanism of action of modafinil (Provigil) is yet to be fully elucidated. It binds to the DAT and requires its presence as well as that of alpha adrenergic receptors, especially alpha 1. In contrast, modafinil does not appear to require the norepinephrine transporter or postsynaptic dopamine receptors. Modafinil's low affinity for the dopamine transporter has led some to question whether its binding there is relevant; however, because plasma levels of modafinil are high, this "compensates" for the low binding affinity. It is believed that the increase in synaptic dopamine following blockade of DAT leads to stimulation of alpha receptors and thus downstream effects on neurotransmitters including glutamate and histamine in wake-promoting regions.

Modafinil can also decrease GABA release in the nucleus accumbens of rats, which can lead to a weak dopaminergic increase, and has also been shown to modulate orexin release, which, in turn, can induce release of both glutamate and histamine in the hypothalamic areas involved in arousal.

Modafinil is typically dosed between 200 and 400 mg/day in a single dose, with a starting dose of 100 mg/day. The most common side effects are headache, nausea, nervousness, anxiety, and insomnia. Despite having some actions on the dopamine system, modafinil does not seem to have much abuse potential and is a Schedule IV drug. [Ballon and Feifel, 2006; Stahl, 2005; Wisor and Eriksson, 2005]

Treating Excessive Sleepiness: Sodium Oxybate

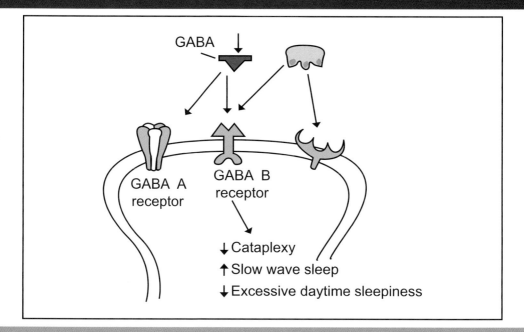

Figure 3.7 Sodium oxybate (Xyrem) is the sodium salt of the endogenous neurochemical gamma-hydroxybutyrate (GHB). It mediates most of its effects at the GHB and $GABA_B$ receptors. GHB can further affect the GABA receptor system through its metabolism to GABA and subsequent actions at $GABA_A$ and $GABA_C$ receptors. Sodium oxybate is also associated with increased serotonin turnover, interactions with endogenous opioids, and possible modulation of dopaminergic activity.

Low-dose sodium oxybate can increase levels of glutamate and dopamine, but at higher doses it reduces levels of these neurotransmitters and increases levels of striatal and mesolimbic serotonin. This is thought to reflect the activation of GHB receptors at low dose and the $GABA_B$ receptors—for which sodium oxybate has only weak affinity—at higher doses.

Sodium oxybate can induce sleep without radically changing the natural sleep pattern and was previously used in general anesthesia. It can consolidate disrupted sleep in people with narcolepsy and also improves the occurrence of cataplexy and other daytime symptoms, however the precise mechanism that is operating to help reduce cataplexy is not fully understood. Sodium oxybate is available as a liquid (0.5 g/mL) and has to be dosed twice nightly: starting dose is 2.25 g/4.5 mL diluted in 2 ounces of water immediately before lying down and again 2.5–4 hours later. Therapeutic total daily dose is generally 6–9 g. Side effects include headache, nausea, dizziness, pain, and somnolence. Sodium oxybate is contraindicated in patients taking sedative hypnotics and in those with succinic semialdehyde dehydrogenase deficiency. For medical use sodium oxybate is Schedule III, although for illicit use it is Schedule I [Maitre, 1997; Lemon et al., 2006]

Treating Excessive Sleepiness: Caffeine

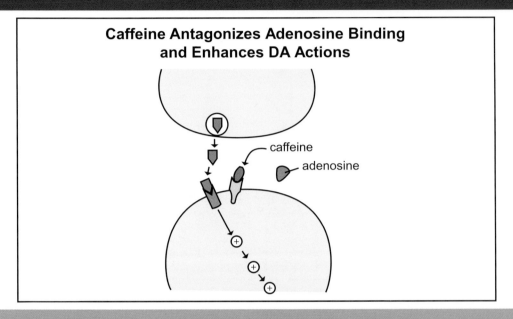

Caffeine Antagonizes Adenosine Binding and Enhances DA Actions

caffeine

adenosine

Figure 3.8 The well known effects of caffeine include enhanced psychomotor vigilance and decreased propensity to sleep, normally at a "dose" of over 150 mg (large cup of coffee). Caffeine works by blocking adenosine -1 (A1) and -2A (A2A) receptors in the basal forebrain, leading to cortical arousal. While the almost ubiquitous A1 receptors are highest in the hippocampus, cerebellum, and some thalamic nuclei, A2A receptors are concentrated in the dopaminergic regions of the brain. A2A and D2 receptors colocalize on GABAergic neurons in the striatum, and stimulation of the A2A receptors by adenosine reduces the affinity of D2 receptors for dopamine, thus, blockade of these receptors by caffeine restores the normal affinity of dopamine for the receptor. Through A1 receptor blockade caffeine can increase levels of cortical acetylcholine release. Caffeine can also increase levels of serotonin, glutamate, and norepinephrine, but the role these actions have in caffeine's effects is not thought to be major.

Wyatt et al. (2004) put a group of 16 subjects on a 'forced desynchrony' protocol where they underwent 28.57-hour wake episodes and 14.28-hour sleep episodes. During the wake condition subjects received either caffeine capsules or a placebo every hour. In the placebo group there were a large number of unintentional sleep onsets especially at the end of wake episodes and following the normal core temperature and melatonin high. In contrast, during the wake episodes the caffeine group showed attenuation of the wake- and circadian-dependent modulation of unintentional sleep onset. The caffeine group also had significantly better results on an addition task, the Digit Symbol Substitution Task, and the Psychomotor Vigilance Task. However, the sleep chances taken by the placebo group meant that on subjective scales of sleepiness this group actually fared better than the caffeine group and, using slow eye movements during wake time as another sign of sleepiness, there was no difference between the groups. Interestingly the caffeine group also showed more impaired sleep during times of normal wakefulness. [Stahl, 2005; Wyatt et al., 2004]

Treatment for Disturbed Sleep: Sleep Aids

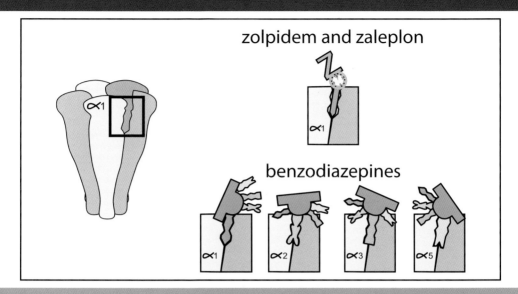

Figure 3.9 There are a number of medications, both prescription and over-the-counter (OTC), that can help improve sleep and thus in turn may reduce excessive sleepiness during waking hours. The classic benzodiazepines bind non-selectively to any of the α-subunit isoforms of GABA$_A$ receptors. This means that, along with their sedative effects, they can also be used for anxiety problems, as muscle relaxants, and as hypnotics. Although these are added benefits for some people, they can lead to problems with next day sedation and psychomotor slowness. In addition, benzodiazepine actions at α5 can lead to memory problems.

The GABA$_A$ modulators zolpidem (Ambien, Ambien CR) and zaleplon (Sonata) show selective affinity for only those GABA$_A$ receptors that include α1 subunits. Thus, although GABA$_A$ modulators and benzodiazepines both act on the same receptors, the newer drugs specifically activate receptors involved in sleep-promoting effects. This more restrictive binding is proposed to be why the drugs have a better safety profile and less tolerance over long-term use. The GABA$_A$ modulators zopiclone (not available in the U.S.) and eszopiclone (Lunesta) may have slightly different mechanism of action, as it is not yet known if they are selective for α1 subunits.

Although sleep aids can be used to improve sleep in some sleep disorders, as well as in psychiatric and medical illnesses, they may not be recommended in all of these disorders. Specific treatment guidelines for several sleep disorders are given on the following pages. [Stahl, in press]

Modulating the Circadian Rhythm: Melatonin

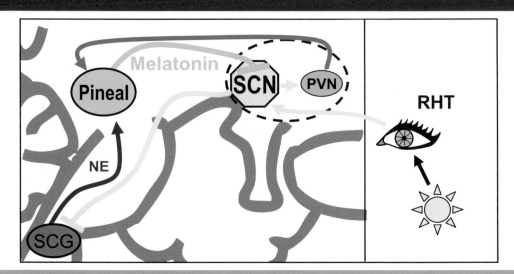

Figure 3.10 Melatonin, an endogenous neurohormone, is a tryptophan/serotonin derivative that is secreted by the pineal gland in increased levels as darkness sets in. It is intimately involved in feelings of tiredness and initiation of sleep. Its synthesis is predominantly controlled by the retinohypothalamic tract (RHT), via the suprachiasmatic nucleus (SCN). From here, the pineal gland can be stimulated either via the paraventricular nucleus (PVN) of the hypothalamus, or via norepinephrine release from the superior cervical ganglion (SCG) in the brainstem/spinal cord, initiated when the SCN is inhibited. The receptors MT1 and MT2 control the relevant actions of melatonin, suppressing neuronal firing and inducing phase shifts respectively. The presence of MT1 receptors in the SCN suggests these mediate sleep-promoting mechanisms.

The general action of melatonin is to reduce sleep onset latency as opposed to maintaining sleep. Although touted as a general sleep-promoting factor, studies show that ingestion of melatonin may only be effective in people whose melatonin levels are low, e.g., night-shift workers or people with insomnia. As such, it can also be used at times when there is not normally melatonin, such as when someone with jet-lag is trying to advance their endogenous circadian rhythm. It has been used additionally to help 'train' people who may be suffering from free-running circadian rhythms such as has been shown in people who are blind.

Synthetic MT1/MT2 agonists, such as ramelteon (Rozerem), have been developed that are around ten times as effective as ingested melatonin for reducing sleep onset latency. Slow-release tablets are being investigated which are able to improve sleep maintenance and duration as well. The effects of these tablets may not be as immediate as other sleep-aids, with several nights administration needed before the full potential is reached. [Pandi-Perumal et al., 2006; Pandi-Perumal et al., 2007]

Treatment Guidelines: Narcolepsy

Drug	Clinical Use	Dose
modafinil	excessive sleepiness	200–400 mg/day
amphetamines	excessive sleepiness	5–60 mg/day*
methylphenidate (d,l)	excessive sleepiness	20–60 mg/day*
sodium oxybate	excessive sleepiness cataplexy	Initially 2.25 g taken just before lying down and again 2.5–4 hours later; usual total daily dose 6–9 g
venlafaxine	cataplexy	37.5–150 mg/day
clomipramine	cataplexy	10–200 mg/day
fluoxetine	cataplexy	20–80 mg/day
protriptyline	cataplexy	5–30 mg/day

*Dosing schedule varies by formulation

Figure 3.11 Management of narcolepsy falls mostly into two categories: drugs for treating excessive sleepiness and drugs for treating cataplexy. Treatment of excessive sleepiness has been discussed in general on previous pages; pharmacologic options and their doses are listed here.

Sodium oxybate has proved useful in the treatment of cataplexy and is the only agent approved for such use. Sodium oxybate is also effective for reducing excessive sleepiness, and additionally may reduce sleep disturbances and improve daytime alertness and concentration.

A number of antidepressants have been used clinically for cataplexy, including tricyclic antidepressants (TCAs), venlafaxine, and fluoxetine, although they have not been studied in large controlled trials. The mechanism for anticataplectic effects is not known, but may be related to their ability to suppress REM sleep. Clomipramine is the most frequently used antidepressant for cataplexy and may also reduce sleep paralysis and hypnagogic hallucinations. Protriptyline is also frequently used, and more recently venlafaxine and fluoxetine as well. Newer antidepressants may not be as efficacious as TCAs, but may be more tolerable.

Although nearly all patients with narcolepsy will require pharmacologic intervention, behavioral management is nonetheless an important part of treatment. It is particularly important for narcolepsy patients to practice good sleep hygiene. These patients should avoid work or lifestyle situations that can cause sleep deprivation or dysregulation, such as shift work, and should not work in hazardous situations. Patients with narcolepsy may benefit from taking brief naps at specified times, which could require coordination with their employers. [Billiard et al., 2006; Stahl, 2005; Thorpy, 2007]

Treatment Guidelines: OSA

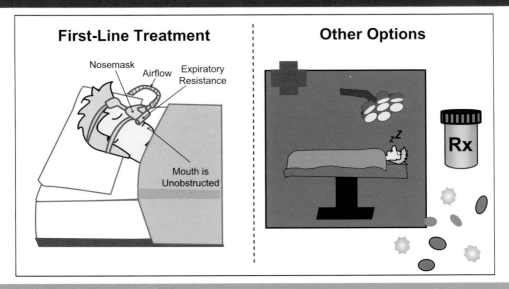

First-Line Treatment

Nosemask
Airflow
Expiratory Resistance
Mouth is Unobstructed

Other Options

Rx

Figure 3.12 The first-line treatment for moderate to severe OSA is continuous positive airway pressure (CPAP). This treatment delivers oxygen through a nose mask while the patient is sleeping so that the upper airway can be kept open. CPAP is very effective at improving sleep quality and reducing sleepiness when used correctly and has the benefit of being effective from the first night's use. However, the apparatus can be uncomfortable for some patients and can lead to problems such as nasal congestion, chest and sinus discomfort, and skin abrasions or rashes where the mask contacts the face. Because of these factors, compliance may be a problem and 20–35% of patients cannot put up with these side effects. Currently in development is a much less irritating nasal cannula which uses warm, humidified air to increase pharyngeal pressure.

Some drug therapies have been used to treat apneas, but are of only marginal benefit. These include protriptyline, which may help by suppressing REM sleep (most apneas occur during REM sleep) as well as by increasing genioglossus muscle tone.

Many patients with apnea experience residual excessive sleepiness, and thus adjunct drug therapy is sometimes necessary. Treatments for excessive sleepiness include modafinil, which is approved for this use, as well as off-label use of methylphenidate and amphetamines. In addition, patients may use caffeine during the day. Sleep aids are not recommended unless the respiratory symptoms are well under control, although Kryger et al. (2007) recently showed in a small study that the melatonin agonist ramelteon reduces sleepiness without negative respiratory effects. Benzodiazepines can exacerbate OSA and are not recommended.

Surgery is an option for people who cannot tolerate CPAP, but may only be successful for those who have obvious anatomical abnormalities in their upper airway. Surgery can include removal of the tonsils, uvula, distal margin of the soft palate, and excessive pharyngeal tissue. More extreme surgery can include tongue reduction or oromaxillofacial surgery. [McGinley et al., 2007; Hirshkowitz and Black, 2007]

Treatment Guidelines: Shift-Work Sleep Disorder

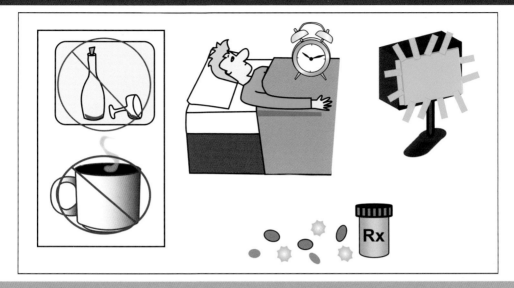

Figure 3.13 Optimizing sleep hygiene for night shift workers is vital. One of the major factors inhibiting sleep is exposure to bright light, which should be counteracted by wearing dark sunglasses on returning home and sleeping in a dark, quiet room. As it is important to try and retrain the core body temperature to the shifted time, the bedroom should be kept cool. A person should refrain from stimulants in the second half of a shift, or a cycle can develop whereby a person who relies on caffeine/tobacco can experience insomnia and then subsequent excessive sleepiness on the next shift. However, strategic use of caffeine early in the shift may be helpful. As light entering the eyes directly affects the hypothalamus, the use of artificial daylight bulbs, known as bright light therapy (BLT), can also be very helpful during the work shift.

Melatonin is useful to help someone phase shift but the degree and direction of shift depends on the time of day it is administered, as melatonin receptor levels are high during the evening and low during the night. When melatonin is administered in the evening the circadian rhythm advances to allow a person to sleep earlier. However, melatonin given early in the morning can cause a phase delay, so that a person will not feel sleepy until later. Hence, against popular thought, it is better to use melatonin for shift-work sleep disorder during the night, at around the normal circadian low of 03:00. Sleep aids can also help with retraining the body to match the shift-work time.

Many of those with shift-work sleep disorder suffer from excessive sleepiness during their wake time. Modafinil is the only currently approved medication for this indication; methylphenidate or amphetamines may be used off-label. [Pandi-Perumal et al., 2006; Czeisler et al., 2005]

Restless Legs Syndrome/ Periodic Limb Movements

Non-pharmacologic Therapy	Pharmacologic Therapy
• Physiotherapy	• DA agonists - ropinirole, pramipexole
• Mild stretching	• DA precursors - l-dopa
• Hot/cold baths	• Sleep aids
• Alerting activities	• Wakefulness aids

• Iron replacement	• Other
	  - gabapentin, opiates,
	    carbamazepine, clonazepam

• Stop other medications	
• Avoid coffee, nicotine, alcohol	

Figure 3.14 For mild RLS, daytime activity and complete abstinence of coffee, alcohol and nicotine is indicated. RLS may also be aggravated by medications including antihistamines, antidopaminergics, and antidepressants, thus the use of these should be investigated and possibly stopped. Various forms of physiotherapy can help, including mild stretching exercises, massage, biofeedback, and leg vibration. RLS, a physical anomaly which may have roots in the brain, may be counteracted by mental activity such as crosswords, video games, stimulating conversation, or painting.

As RLS is thought to involve problems with iron storage/metabolism, long-term supplementation can be very effective, more so than one high dose of iron dextran.

Ropinirole and pramipexole significantly reduce motor and sleep disturbances and are both approved to treat RLS. Their side effects can include nausea, dizziness, vomiting, constipation, fatigue and somnolence. Ropinirole is given 1–3 hours before bedtime at an initial dose of 0.25 mg, which can be increased up to 4 mg/night on a slow titration schedule. Pramipexole is given 2–3 hours before bedtime at an initial dose of 0.125 mg, which can be increased after 4–7 days to 0.25 mg and then again to 0.5 mg.

Also effective may be the dopamine precursor l-dopa, which is approved in some European countries in combination with benserazide, a dopa decarboxylase inhibitor that prevents conversion of l-dopa to dopamine in the periphery.

For PLMs, anticonvulsants such as gabapentin or benzodiazepines including clonazepam may reduce muscle contractions in some people, the latter being the most widely used drug for this condition. Also used is the GABA agonist baclofen, which can inhibit release of neurotransmitters that stimulate muscle contractions. [Vignatelli et al., 2006; Silber et al., 2004]

Summary

One of the easiest, earliest ways to try and help a patient with excessive sleepiness is to investigate if poor sleep/wake hygiene is adding to excessive sleepiness problems.

Medications can be used both to treat excessive sleepiness during waking hours and help alleviate sleep problems which can also lead to excessive sleepiness.

Wake-promoting agents include modafinil, amphetamines, and methylphenidate.

Specific treatments for specific disorders include sodium oxybate for narcolepsy, CPAP for OSA, and dopamine agonists for RLS/PLMs.

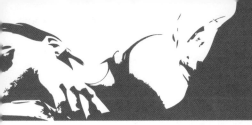

American Academy of Sleep Medicine. The International Classification of Sleep Disorders, revised: diagnostic and coding manual. Chicago, Illinois; 2001.

Arnsten AFT and Li B-M. Neurobiology of executive functions: catecholamine influences on prefrontal cortical functions. Biol Psychiatry 2005;57:1377-84.

Ballon JS and Feifel D. A systematic review of modafinil: potential clinical uses and mechanisms of action. J Clin Psychiatry 2006;67:4.

Barger LK, Cade BE, Ayas NT et al. Extended work shifts and the risk of motor vehicle crashes among interns. NEJM 2005;352:125-34.

Billiard M et al. EFNS guidelines on management of narcolepsy. Eur J Neurology 2006;13:1035-48.

Buckley TM and Schatzberg AF. On the interactions of the hypothalamic-pituitary-adrenal (HPA) axis and sleep: normal HPA axis activity and circadian rhythm, exemplary sleep disorders. J Clin Endocrinol Metab. 2005;90:3106-14.

Czeisler CA et al. Modafinil for excessive sleepiness associated with shift-work sleep disorder. N Engl J Med. 2005;353:476-86.

Dijk D-J and Lockley SW. Functional Genomics of Sleep and Circadian Rhythm. Invited review: integration of human sleep-wake regulation and circadian rhythmicity. J Appl Physiol 2002;92:862-62.

Dinges DF, Pack F, Williams K, et al. Cumulative sleepiness, mood disturbance, and psychomotor vigilance performance decrements during a week of sleep restricted to 4-5 hours per night. Sleep. 1997;20:267-77.

Drake C, Nickel C, Burduvali E, Roth T, et al. The Pediatric Daytime Sleepiness Scale (PDSS): sleep habits and school outcomes in middle-school children. Sleep 2003;26:455-58.

Drummond SPA, Meloy MJ Mathew A et al. Compensatory recruitment after sleep deprivation and the relationship with performance. Psychiatry Res: Neuroimmaging 2005;140:211-23.

Erman MK. Selected sleep disorders: restless legs syndrome and periodic limb movement disorder, sleep apnea syndrome, and narcolepsy. Psychiatr Clin North Am. 2006;29:947-67.

Gilmartin GS, Daly RW and Thomas RJ. Recognition and management of complex sleep-disordered breathing. Curr Opin Pulm Med. 2005;11:485-93.

Heyder K, Suchan B and Daum I. Cortico-subcortical contributions to executive control. Acta Psychologica 2004;115:271-89.

Hirshkowitz M and Black J. Effect of adjunctive modafinil on wakefulness and quality of life in patients with excessive sleepiness-associated obstructive sleep apnoea/hypopnoea syndrome. CNS Drugs 2007;21:407-16.

Horne J and Reyner L. Vehicle accidents related to sleep: a review. Occup Environ Med 1999;56:289-94.

Lemon MD, Strain JD, Farver DK. Sodium oxybate for cataplexy. Ann Pharmacother 2006;40:433-40.

Maitre M. The y-hydroxybutyrate signaling system in brain: organization and functional implications. Prog Neurobiol 1997;51:337-61.

McGinley BM et al. A nasal cannula can be used to treat obstructive sleep apnea. Am J Respir Crit Care Med 2007;176:194-200.

Meir H et al. Chapter 50: Use of Clinical Tools and Tests in Sleep Medicine in Principles and Practice of Sleep Medicine, 4th Edition. Elsevier; 2005,

Mistlberger, RE. Circadian regulation of sleep in mammals: role of the suprachiasmatic nucleus. Brain Res Brain Res Rev 2005;49:429-454.

Pandi-Perumal SR et al. Melatonin. Nature's most versatile biological signal? FEBS Journal 2006;273:2813-38.

Pandi-Perumal SR et al. Drug insight: the use of melatonergic agonists for the treatment of insomnia – focus on ramelteon. Nature Neurology 2007;3:221-28.

Sangal RB, Thomas L and Mitler MM. Maintenance of wakefulness test and multiple sleep latency test. Measurement of different abilities in patients with sleep disorders. Chest 1992;101:898-902.

Saper CB, Lu J, Chou TC and Gooley J. The hypothalamic integrator for circadian rhythms. TINS 2005;28:152-157.

Scammell TE. The neurobiology, diagnosis and treatment of narcolepsy. Ann Neurol 2003;53:154-66.

Schwartz JR and Roth T. Shift work sleep disorder: burden of illness and approaches to management. Drugs. 2006;66:2357-70.

Shipp S. The brain circuitry of attention. TICS 2004;8:223-30.

Silber MH et al. An algorithm for the management of restless legs syndrome. Mayo Clin Proc. 2004 Jul;79(7):916-22. Erratum in: Mayo Clin Proc 2004;79:1341.

Sleep Foundation 2005 'Sleep in America Poll' http://www.sleep-solutions.com/phys/education/NSF_2005_Sleep_in_America_Poll_Results.htm

Stahl SM. Essential psychopharmacology 3rd Ed. New York, NY: Cambridge University Press; in press.

Stahl SM. Illustrated insights in sleep: excessive sleepiness. San Diego, CA: NEI Press; 2005.

Stenberg D. Neuroanatomy and neurochemistry of sleep. Cell Mol Life Sci 2007;64:1187-1204.

Suzuki K, Ohida T, Kaneita Y et al. Daytime sleepiness, sleep habits and occupational accidents among hospital nurses. J Adv Nurs 2005;52:445-53.

Thomas RJ et al. Functional imaging of working memory in obstructive sleep-disordered breathing. J Appl Physiol 2005;98:2226-34.

Thorpy M. Therapeutic advances in narcolepsy. Sleep Med 2007;8(4):427-40.

Vignatelli L et al. EFNS guidelines on management of restless legs syndrome and periodic limb movement disorder in sleep. Eur J Neurology 2006;13:1049-65.

Wisor JP, Eriksson KS. Dopaminergic-adrenergic interactions in the wake promoting mechanism of modafinil. Neurosci 2005;132:1027-34.

Wyatt JK et al. Low-dose repeated caffeine administration for circadian-phase-dependent performance degradation during extended wakefulness. Sleep 2004;27:374-11.

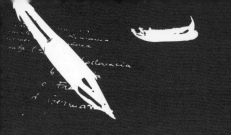
To receive your certificate of CME credit or participation, please complete the posttest and activity evaluation answer sheet found on the next page and return by postage-paid mail or fax it to 760-931-8713. Upon receipt, your posttest will be graded and, along with your certificate (if a score of 70% or higher was attained), returned to you by mail. Alternatively, you may complete these items online and immediately print your certificate at **www.neiglobal. com/pt/07sleepwakemonograph.**

1. Most wake circuits originate in the
   A. Thalamus
   B. Brainstem arousal nuclei (BAN)
   C. Hypothalamus
   D. Basal forebrain

2. Increases in cortisol release can lead to
   A. Hyperarousal
   B. Hypoarousal

3. The peak time for sleep-related vehicular accidents is:
   A. 02:00–06:00
   B. 14:00–16:00
   C. 10:00–12:00
   D. A and B
   E. B and C

4. The instruction, "Lie quietly in a comfortable position, keep your eyes closed, and try to fall asleep" is part of the:
   A. Maintenance of Wakefulness Test
   B. Multiple Sleep Latency Test
   C. Epworth Sleepiness Scale

5. Orexin/hypocretin neurons are only found in a small population of cells in the:
   A. Thalamus
   B. Hypothalamus
   C. Hippocampus
   D. Locus coeruleus

6. Melatonin is released from the brainstem.
   A. True
   B. False

7. Which statement is right?
   A. All of those with restless legs syndrome have concurrent periodic limb movements
   B. All of those with periodic limb movements have concurrent restless legs syndrome
   C. People with periodic limb movements do not necessarily have restless legs syndrome
   D. Periodic limb movements and restless legs syndrome never occur together

8. Sodium oxybate can be converted into:
   A. Dopamine
   B. Glutamate
   C. Norepinephrine
   D. GABA

9. CPAP for obstructive sleep apnea is an acronym that stands for:
   A. Concentrated positive airway pressure
   B. Continuous positive airway pressure
   C. Continuous positive alveolar pressure
   D. Concentrated pressure and presence

Diagnosis and Treatment of Sleep/Wake Disorders
Posttest

To receive your certificate of CME credit or participation, please complete the posttest and activity evaluation answer sheet found on this page and return by postage-paid mail or fax it to 760-931-8713. Upon receipt, your posttest will be graded and, along with your certificate (if a score of 70% or higher was attained), returned to you by mail. Alternatively, you may complete these items online and immediately print your certificate at **www.neiglobal.com/pt/07sleepwakemonograph.** (Circle the correct answer)

Answer Sheet

1. A	B	C	D		6. A	B			
2. A	B				7. A	B	C	D	
3. A	B	C	D	E	8. A	B	C	D	
4. A	B	C			9. A	B	C	D	
5. A	B	C	D						

Activity Evaluation: Please rate the following, using a scale of:

1-poor	2-fair	3-good	4-very good	5-excellent

1. The overall quality of the content was…   1 2 3 4 5

2. The relevance of the content to my professional needs was…   1 2 3 4 5

3. The level at which the learning objective was met of teaching me to recognize underlying causes of sleep/wake disorders   1 2 3 4 5

4. The level at which the learning objective was met of teaching me to identify patients for whom direct treatment of sleep/wake problems is necessary   1 2 3 4 5

5. The level at which the learning objective was met of teaching me to effectively implement treatment plans for patients with sleep/wake disorders   1 2 3 4 5

6. The level at which this activity was objective, scientifically balanced, and free of commercial bias was…   1 2 3 4 5

7. The overall quality of this activity was…   1 2 3 4 5

8. Based on my experience and knowledge, the level of this activity was:

   Too Basic   Basic   Appropriate   Complex   Too Complex

9. Based on the information presented in this activity, I will:
   A. Change my practice
   B. Seek additional information on this topic
   C. Do nothing as current practice reflects activity's recommendations
   D. Do nothing as the content was not convincing

10. What barriers might keep you from implementing changes in your practice you'd like to make as a result of participating in this activity?

11. The following additional information about this topic would help me in my practice:

12. How could this activity have been improved?

Name: _____ Credentials: _____

Specialty: _____

Address: _____

City, State, Zip: _____

Email: _____ Phone: _____

NEUROSCIENCE EDUCATION INSTITUTE
CME DEPARTMENT
1930 Palomar Point Way, Suite 101
Carlsbad, CA 92008

BUSINESS REPLY MAIL

FIRST-CLASS MAIL   PERMIT NO. 1323   CARLSBAD, CA

POSTAGE WILL BE PAID BY ADDRESSEE

NEUROSCIENCE EDUCATION INSTITUTE
1930 PALOMAR POINT WAY STE 101
CARLSBAD CA 92008-9558